Pandemic Flu Planning
in Africa
Thoughts from a Nigerian Case Study

Cheryl Loeb, Lynn McGrath, and Sudhir Devalia

Center for Technology and National Security Policy
National Defense University

August 2009

Sudhir Devalia is a Research Associate at the Nati onal Defense University's Center for Technology and National Security Policy, wh ere he has conducted research on various aspects of African security. Previously, he served as a T reasury Officer in Zam bia for Finance Bank Ltd., and a Financial Advisor at Investor's Group, a financial planning company in Montreal, Canada. Mr. Devalia holds a Master of Arts in Inte rnational Commerce and Policy from George Mason University.

Cheryl Loeb is a Research Associate at the Center for Technology and National Security Policy at the National Defense University and is also a Ph.D. candidate in the Public and International Affairs program at George Ma son University. At CTNSP Ms. Loeb works on health security and biological weapons pro liferation threats. She may be contacted via email at loebc@ndu.edu or by phone at (202) 685-2397.

Lynn McGrath Jr. is a Research Associate at th e Center for Technology and National Security Policy. His research in terests include medical diplomacy, disaster relief operations, and innovative use of technology in the military and medical fields. He holds a Bachelors degree in Neuroscience from Dartmouth College and will pursue a m edical degree at the University of Central Florida.

Acknowledgements: CTNSP would like to acknowledge the exceptional work of North American Management and the project team who developed and administered the pandemic influenza planning course in Nigeria under contract to CTNSP. Their hard work resulted in a very successful course that was lauded by all participants involved. The essence of their work is captured in pages 12-16 of this paper.

Defense & Technology Papers are published by the National Defense University Center for Technology and National Security Policy, Fort Lesley J. McNair, Washington, DC. CTNSP publications are available online at http://www ndu.edu/ctnsp/publications html.

Contents

Introduction

Over the past 35 years, dozens of new and fr ightening diseases ha ve been iden tified, among them hepatitis C virus, Ebola and ot her hemorrhagic viruses, Legionnaires' disease, Nipah encephalitis, H5N1 inf luenza, SARS, the new arenav irus Lujo, which causes hemorrhagic fever in its victim s, and, m ost pervasively, the hum an immunodeficiency virus (HIV/AIDS). The emergence of H5N1 avian flu in 1996, coupled with the recent declaration of an H1N1 influenza pandem ic, demonstrate the urgent need for countries to have pandem ic preparedness plans in place. For nations that are unprepared, a pandem ic could result in devastating so cial, economic, and health consequences, including a high number of fat alities. Nowhere is this more so the case than in countries with underdeveloped health care systems.

The potential im pact of a severe pandem ic requires that nations throughout the w orld develop pandemic response plans before the ons et of disease. Mainta ining continuity of operations and protecting a nati ons' greatest asset, its peop le, during a pandem ic requires developing effective plans before a pande mic becomes severe. These plans need to include such key issu es as iden tification of roles and r esponsibilities, infection control, the identification of health care facilities, maintaining security, providing logistical support for food, m edicine, and other comm odities, communication procedures, and developing and distributing vaccines and antivirals.

In recognition of the loom ing threat of an influenza p andemic, North Am erican Management, under contract to the Center for Technology and National Security Policy (CTNSP), developed and administered a program to help build pandemic influenza crisis-response capacities. We held an Avian In fluenza/Pandemic Influenza Policy P lanning workshop in Nigeria in June 2007 with the objective of assisting selected Nigerian officials in evaluating their nation's pandemic response plan. After assessing the viability of the Nigerian National Integrated Avian a nd Pandemic Influenza Plan, a number of key action items for various Nigerian ministries were suggested. These action items would act to strengthen not only interagency comm unication and cooperation, but also the pandemic response in the country.

The importance of further pandem ic planning in Nigeria and neighboring countries cannot be understated. The current H1N1 out break, characterized at th e time of writing by the World Health Organization as moderately severe, still has the po tential to mutate and become much more deadly, necessitating the urgent need for pandemic planning.

The recently established U.S. Africa Comm and, in partnership with the United State s Agency for International Development (USAID), Pacific Comm and, and other international partners, has developed a Pandemic Response Program aimed at strengthening partner nations' military capacities to plan for, and respond to, pandem ics. The development of both m ilitary and civ ilian pandemic response p lans in Africa, through the partnership of AFRICOM and othe r international part ners, is vital in preparing for a severe pandemic and mitigating its consequences.

Epidemics and Pandemics in Human History

"After gasping for several hours they becam e delirious and … many died struggling to clear their airways of a blood-tinged froth that sometimes gushed from their nose and mouth. It was a dreadful business."
--Isaac Starr, 3rd year medical student, University of Pennsylvania, 1918[1]

There are many crises that one can im agine could lead to chaos—but perhaps none have the potential to affect each m ember of a society as profoundly as a pandem ic.[2] Infectious disease knows no boundary, particularly one that is capable of hum an-to-human transmission, such as sm allpox or influenza. As history has shown, a large outbreak of communicable disease can cause mass m orbidity and mortality, resulting in severe social and economic disruption.

In his *History of the Peloponnesian War*, Thucydides wrote about a "plague" that struck the city of Athens in the summer of 430 B. C.E. Occurring early in the Peloponnesian war, the epidemic lasted until 427 B.C.E. and is believed to have killed 25 to 35 percent of the Athenian population.[3] The outbreak of disease cau sed "a serious breakdow n in respect for laws and social norms ….and that may in turn have played a longer-range role in what m any scholars have si nce seen as a col lapse of At henian morality during and after the Peloponnesian War."[4] The "plague" described by Thucydides has never been identified but is believed to have been either smallpox or measles.

The first recorded large-scale outbreak of bubonic plague, known as the Plague of Justinian, occurred in 541, kill ing thousands of people in Constantinople, Egypt, and elsewhere along the eastern Med iterranean, reaching as far as Italy and Tunisia by 54 4. J.N. Hays, in *Epidemics and Pandemics: Their Impact on Human History,* describes the tumultuous effects the plague had on society:

> Witnesses agreed that the immediate effect of the se plague visitations was catastrophic. Social confusion and econom ic paralysis resulted. All work ceased. Shops closed for lack of workers and customers. Fields were abandoned, crops remained unharvested, fruits fell rott en to the gr ound, and fl ocks and her ds wandered untended in fields and pastures. Elite members of society remained unburied when their servants predeceased them.[5]

The second major outbreak of bubonic plague, known then as the Black Death, appeared in 1346. Spread by the bite of infected fleas, it swept rapidly throughout Europe and Asia

---

[1] Isaac Starr, "Influenza in 1918: Recollections of the Epidemic in Philadelphia," *Annals of Internal Medicine,* 2006;145:13–140, available at <http://www.annals.org/cgi/reprint/145/2/138.pdf>.
[2] Pandemics, an epidemic of infectious disease that spreads across a large population, often globally, are quite rare, generally occurring only 2–3 times a century or less.
[3] J.N. Hays, *Epidemics and Pandemics: Their Impact on Human History* (Santa Barbara, CA: ABC-CLIO, Inc, 2005).
[4] Ibid.
[5] Ibid., 27.

along maritime trade routes, killing between 30 and 40 percent of populations infected (some estimates are as high as 60 percent). Poor sanitation and severe overcrowding in cities further led to the rapid spread of disease. Small outbreaks of bubonic plague continued to reappear in some locations until 1667. According to one author, prior to the outbreak of plague, population levels in Europe were at such a height that the economic and social situation reflected "a world of labor surplus, land shortage, and food shortage—low wages, high rents, and high prices."[6] Perversely, the outbreak of plague in Europe eventually brought higher wages and a better standard of living for the survivors due to the large number of human casualties from the disease.

Pandemic Influenza

The single deadliest outbreak of disease in the 20th century, and perhaps all of human history, was the 1918–1919 influenza pandemic. The outbreak of Spanish Flu, as it came to be called, occurred in late winter and early spring of 1918, with mild cases of the flu appearing sporadically around the globe. Beginning in August 1918, near the end of World War I, a second, more virulent, wave of the virus began appearing, spreading rapidly along trade and military troop deployment routes. Efforts to stop the spread of the disease were severely hampered by a lack of medical supplies and a severe shortage of healthcare workers healthy enough to care for those infected with the influenza virus. Hospitals were quickly overfilled with the sick and dying, and morgues were unable to deal with the large influx of corpses.[7] During the epidemic, many cities enforced social distancing restrictions, closing schools and banning large public gatherings in an effort to stem the tide of infection, to no avail.

While the second wave of the influenza outbreak began declining worldwide by the end of December 1918, some countries experienced a third and final wave of the disease in January and February 1919. Within the space of a year the Spanish flu virus killed an estimated 50 million people worldwide (some estimates have placed the number as high as 100 million).[8]

---

[6] Ibid., 48.

[7] John M. Barry, *The Great Influenza: The Epic Story of the Deadliest Plague in History* (New York: Penguin Books, 2004).

[8] "Influenza research at the human and animal interface," WHO Working Group Report, 21-22 September, 2006, available at <http://www.who.int/csr/resources/publications/influenza/ WHO_CDS _EPR _GIP _2006_3C.pdf>.

Understanding Influenza Viruses

Influenza viruses are class ified as type A, B, or C, base d on their protein composition. Type A viruses are found in m any kinds of anim als, including ducks, chickens, pigs, and humans. Type A is the most common and typically causes the most serious epidem ics and pandem ics in hum ans. Type A viruses are subdivided into groups based on two surface proteins: Hemagglutinin (HA) and Ne uraminidase (NA). Scientists have characterized 16 HA subtypes and 9 NA subtypes. Scientists have identified the 1918-1919 pandemic causing virus as an H1N1 type A virus.

Source: Jeffrey K. Taubenberger and David M. Morens, "1918 Influenza: The Mother of all Pandemics," *Emerging Infectious Diseases*, January 2006, available at <http://www.cdc.gov/ncidod/eid/vol12no01/05-0979.htm>.

Two more flu pandem ics occurred in the 20 [th] century. T he 1957 flu (H2N2 type A influenza), named the Asian flu for w here cases were first identified, caused roughly two million deaths worldwide and abo ut 69,800 d eaths in the United States. [9] The third pandemic was first detected in Hong K ong in 1968. The Hong Kong influenza (H3N2 type A influenza) resulted in less than one million deaths worldwide, with roughly 34,000 deaths in the United States (t his is roughly equal to the num ber of mortalities that occur in the United States during the annual seasonal flu).

H5N1 –Avian Influenza

In 1996, epidemiologists discovered an entirely new variety of type A influenza, known as subtype H5N1, whe n it was first isolat ed from a farmed goose in Guangdong, China. In 1997, a m assive outbreak of H5N1 avia n influenza occurred in Hong Kong poultry markets, resulting in 18 cases of bird-to-hum an transmission of the virus and six deaths. A rapid cu lling of over 1.5 m illion birds in ju st three days is though t to have averted further transmission of the virus.[10]

Since the initial outbreak of avian influenza in poultry and hum ans in Hong Kong in 1997, there have been hundreds of cases of hu man infections throughout the world. As of September 24, 2009, the W orld Health Organi zation (WHO) reported that there have been 442 human cases of H5N1 reported in 15 countries, 262 of which have been fatal. [11] H5N1 outbreaks have led to m ass culling of in fected bird populations, increased disease surveillance, including passenger screen ing at airpo rts, vaccine and antivira l development, and pandemic response planning.

---

[9] U.S. Department of Health and Human Services, "Pandemics and Pandemic Scares in the 20th Century," February 12, 2004, available at <http://www.hhs.gov/nvpo/pandemics/flu3.htm>.
[10] World Health Organization, "H5N1 avian influenza: Timeline of major events," March 23, 2009, available at <http://www.who.int/csr/disease/avian_influenza/Timeline_09_03_23.pdf>.
[11] World Health Organization, "Cumulative Number of Confirmed Human Cases of Avian Influenza A/(H5N1) Reported to WHO," September 24, 2009, available at <http://www.who.int/csr/disease/avian_influenza/country/cases_table_2009_09_24/en/index html>.

In light of the potential threat of an H5 N1 pandemic, the World Health Organization launched an influenza tracking system , is working on the developm ent of new recombinant H5N1 vaccine viruses, and has developed guidance documents on infection control, diagnosis and treatm ent, disease surveillance, and laboratory procedures for detection of H5N1 virus, to name a few.[12]

H1N1 Pandemic Influenza

In early April 2009, reports began to surface in Mexico of an unusual outbreak of disease. Patients began showing up at hospitals sym ptomatic with fever, cough, vomiting, and, in some patients, acute respiratory infections and pneumonia. In late April, the U.S. Centers for Disease Control activated its Em ergency Operations Center when cases of the disease appeared in California, where scien tists identified it as nov el A in fluenza virus, H1N1. On April 26, with cases of H1N1 identified in Canada, Mexico, and the United States, the United States Governm ent declared a pub lic health emergency, which allowed for the rapid shipment of the antivirals Ta miflu and Relenza from the strategic national stockpile.

The spread of H1N1 prom pted the World H ealth Organization to declare the outbreak a pandemic on June 11, 2009:

> Globally, we have good reason to believe that this pandem ic, at least in its early days, will be of moderate severity. As we know from experience, severity can vary, depending on m any factors, from one country to another. On presen t evidence, the overwhelm ing majority of patients experience mild symptoms and make a rapid and full recover y, often in the absence of any form of medical treatment.[13]

The WHO ranks pandemics in six levels (the WHO phases refer to the geographic spread of the virus vice the severity of it):

- Phase 1: no viruses circulating among ani mals have been reported to cause infections in humans.

- Phase 2: an anim al influenza virus ci rculating among domesticated or wild animals is known to have caused inf ection in humans, and is therefore considered a potential pandemic threat.

- Phase 3: an animal or hum an-animal influenza reassortment virus has caused sporadic cases or sm all clusters of disease in people, but has not resulted in human-to-human transmission sufficient to sustain community-level outbreaks. Limited human-to-human transmission may occur under some circumstances.

---

[12] World Health Organization, "Pandemic (H1N1) 2009 briefing note 3 (revised)," July 16, 2009, available at <http://www.who.int/csr/disease/swineflu/notes/h1n1_surveillance_20090710/en/index.html>.
[13] Margaret Chan, World Health Organization, "World now at start of 2009 influenza pandemic," June 11, 2009, available at <http://www.who.int/mediacentre/news/statements/2009/ h1n1_pandemic_phase6_20090611/en/index html>.

- Phase 4: is characterized by verified hum an-to-human transmission of an anim al or human-animal influenza reassortm ent virus able to cau se "community-level outbreaks."

- Phase 5: is characterized by human-to-human spread of the virus into at le ast two countries in one WHO region. W hile most countries will n ot be affected at this stage, the declaration of Phase 5 is a strong signal that a pandem ic is imm inent and that the time to finalize the organization, communication, and implementation of the planned mitigation measures is short.

- Phase 6: is the pandem ic phase. It is ch aracterized by community level outbreaks in at least one other country in a different WHO region in addition to the criteria defined in Phase 5. Designation of this pha se will indicate that a global pandemic is under way.[14]

Pandemic Severity Index

The U.S. Centers for Disease Control and Pr evention has also developed a five-level pandemic severity index (PSI), sim ilar to the system for categorizing hurricanes. The proposed PSI has five di fferent categories of pandem ics. Category 1 represents moderate severity and category 5 represents the m ost severe. The severity of a pandemic is primarily determined by the case fatality rate, or percentage of infected people who die. A category 1 pandem ic is as harmful as a s evere seasonal influenza season, while a pandem ic with the sam e intensity of the 1918 flu pandem ic, or worse, would be classified as category 5.

Source: U.S. Department of Health and Human Services, "HHS Unveils Two New Efforts to Advance Pandemic Flu Preparedness," February 1, 2007, available at <http://www.hhs.gov/news/press/2007pres/ 20070201 html>.

By October 17, 2009, the WHO ha d reported mo re than 414,000 laboratory confirm ed cases of H1N1 influenza infections , and 5,000 confirm ed deaths worldwide.[15] However, as many countries have stopped counting individual cases, the actual case count is likely significantly higher, with some estimates in the millions of cases worldwide.

Scientists and health o fficials will continu e to m onitor the disease as the Northern hemisphere enters its annual influenza season. T here is a potential for the virus to m utate during this tim e and re-em erge at a later date, causing a much m ore severe form of disease. This is due to processe s called antigenic drift and antigen ic shift. In antig enic

---

[14] World Health Organization, "Current WHO phase of pandemic alert," available online at <http://www.who.int/csr/disease/avian_influenza/phase/en/>.

[15] World Health Organization, "Pandemic (H1N1) 2009 –Update 71,) October 17, 2009, available at <http://www.who.int/csr/don/2009_10_23/en/index.html>.

drift, gradual changes occur th rough point mutations in two m ain surface proteins, hemagglutinin and neuram inidase. These m utations can cause m inor changes to the surface proteins, resulting in new v irus strains that may not be recogn ized by antibo dies developed in response to previous influenza strains. [16] Antigenic shift refers to an abr upt, major change that produces a novel influenza A virus that was not previously circulating in humans. This can occur through direct animal-to-human transmission or through mixing of hum an influenza A and anim al influenza A virus g enes. In th is case, individuals are unlikely to ha ve antibodies from previous influenza strains, m aking the population more susceptible to infection.[17]

Given pandemic influenza's potential to cause massive loss of life (if, in f act, the virus goes through antigenic shift), it is important that a nation have in place a proper action plan to p rotect its p eople and en sure the continuity of operati ons essential to the maintenance of a viable state. W hile the im portance of U.S. dom estic preparedness is obvious, the nature of a pandem ic requires that we also consider the implications for our national security of poorly prep ared nations abroad. As the former Director General of the WHO, Gro Harlem Brundtland has stated, "in a globalize d world, we all swim in a single microbial sea."[18]

---

[16] Centers for Disease Control and Prevention, "Influenza Viruses," November 18, 2005, available at <http://www.cdc.gov/flu/avian/gen-info/flu-viruses htm>.

[17] Ibid.

[18] Brundtland, G.H, "Address to the Codex Alimentarius Commission meeting," July 2-7, 2001.

Health in Africa

Few places on earth demonstrate the devastating effects widespread disease can have on a society as clearly as Africa. Indeed, in sub- Saharan Africa, more than 60 percent of all deaths are due to infectious disease.[19] Outbreaks of cholera and Ebola occur frequently in Africa, and HIV and m alaria are endem ic throughout the contin ent. In 2006 alone, malaria was declared endem ic in 45 countries in Africa, with ove r 212 million cases and roughly 800,000 deaths, 91 percent of which we re in children under 5 years of age. [20] In urban areas the danger is exacerbated by popul ation density, unsanitary living conditions, and unhygienic water sources. In Zim babwe, for example, from August 2008 to June 2009, 98,000 cases of cholera and over 4,000 deaths were reported that were attributable to unsanitary living conditions and lack of medical care.[21]

African countries have to deal with m any diseases, and wid espread poverty means that they are les s able to combat them. At the personal level this m eans inability to a fford such necessities as household cleaning products, soap, and m osquito nets. It can also mean a village farmer refusing to cull protein-rich poultry in an avian influenza outbreak, or a patient unable to afford vaccines, antiv irals, or other prophylactics. At the national level, a lack of government funds has meant a reduction in capacity of the health care and education sectors. In the health care sector this has led to fewer clinics with fewer beds, and outdated medical equipment run by underpaid medical staff. For every 10,000 people in the Democratic Republic of Congo (a hotbe d for disease due to its tropical clim ate), only eight hospital beds and one physician ar e available, compared to 31 beds and 26 physicians in the United States. [22] Due to a lack of funding, few governm ent-subsidized medicines are av ailable and tran sport and infrastructure weaknesses ham per their distribution to remote areas.

A dearth in the education secto r has similar consequences. Fewer schools and a low standard of education have led to entire populations unable to understand what HIV is and how it is transm itted.[23] Locally educated doctors and nurses have learned their trade in educational institutions lim ited by lack of both equipm ent and skilled professors, making available treatment basic in na ture, and research and developm ent on pharmaceuticals almost non-existent. During th e 2008 outbreak of the "Lujo virus" in South Africa, for exam ple, an infected indivi dual in Zambia could not be treated for the disease and had to be airlifted to South Africa for treatment, resulting in f our deaths in

---

[19]The Global Health Council, "The Impact of Infectious Diseases," available at <http://www.globalhealth.org/infectious_diseases/>.

[20] Global Malaria Partnership, "Key malaria facts," 2008, available at <http://www.rollbackmalaria.org/keyfacts.html>.

[21] World Health Organization, "Cholera in Zimbabwe: Update 4," June 9, 2009, available at <http://www.who.int/csr/don/2009_06_09/en/index.html>.

[22] World Health Organization, "World Health Statistics 2009: Health workforce, infrastructure, essential medicines," available at <http://www.who.int/whosis/whostat/EN_WHS09_Table6.pdf>.

[23] In a 2006 rape trial, now-President Jacob Zuma of South Africa admitted having unprotected sex with his HIV-positive accuser, saying he showered afterwards to stop infection. More information available at <http://www.nytimes.com/2006/05/08/world/africa/08cnd-africa.html?scp=6&sq=zuma%20hiv&st=cse>.

both countries. The identification of the viru s and all genetic tes ting was done in the United States as neither African country had the means to do so.[24]

African countries unable to cope with hea lth issues are further burdened by the high prevalence of HIV in their populations. The average life expectancy in many sub-Saharan African countries has plumm eted in recent ye ars, leaving even relatively prosperous countries such as South Africa with a life expectancy of just 49 years because of an HIV prevalence of over 18 percent. [25] In 2007, sub-Saharan Africa, which is hom e to 12 percent of the world's population, accounted fo r two-thirds of the wor ld's HIV-positive population, an estim ated 22 m illion cases.[26] HIV has caused a contraction in hum an capital, a shortage of teacher s and doctors, and a surge of orphans that governments can not support. It has afflic ted African societies from the remotest of villages to the highest echelons of society and has caused a "hollowin g out" effect that has weakened ess ential state infrastructures, priming states for internal collapse and regional conflict.

Highly Virulent H5N1 Avian Influenza in Africa

Our early research on pandemic influenza planning took place in Nigeria. Highly pathogenic H5N1 was first detected in chicke ns in the northern Nige rian state of Ka duna in January 2006. H5N1 quickly sp read to 25 of 26 Nigerian st ates and led to the culling of roughly 368,000 domestic birds.[27]

Nigeria acts as th e wintering area for the garganey (*Anas querquedula*), the most numerous waterfowl species m igrating between Africa and Eurasia. [28] In a study investigating the im pact of m igration routes for Nigeria, the CDC found that "the wintering area in Nigeria where this duck was c aught and remained for 8 weeks be fore spring migration is located where a large num ber of outbreaks have occurred repeatedly since February 2006."[29]

Scientists now believe that som e migratory waterfowl, carrying the H5N1 virus, have travelled along their traditional m igratory routes and introduced H5N1 influenza to various poultry flocks, thus spreading the di sease across long distances and introducing it to new populations (see figur e 1). In m id-2005, for example, more than 6,000 m igratory

---

[24] Thomas Briese, et al, "Genetic Detection and Characterization of Lujo Virus, a New Hemorrhagic Fever-Associated Arenavirus in Southern Africa," *PLoS Pathogens*, May 2009, available at <http://www.plospathogens.org/article/info%3Adoi%2F10.1371%2Fjournal.ppat.1000455>.

[25] Central Intelligence Agency, "World Fact Book: South Africa," available at <https://www.cia.gov/ library/publications/the-world-factbook/geos/sf.html>.

[26] UNAIDS, "2008 Report on the Global Aids Epidemic: Annex HIV and AIDS estimates and data, 2007 and 2001," 2008, available online at <http://data.unaids.org/pub/GlobalReport/2008/jc1510 _2008_global_report_pp211_234_en.pdf>.

[27] Fusaro A, Joannis T, Monne I, Salviato A, Yakubu B, Meseko C, et al, "Introduction into Nigeria of a distinct genotype of avian influenza virus (H5N1)," *Emerging Infectious Disease,* March 2009, available at <http://www.cdc.gov/EID/content/15/3/445.htm>.

[28] Gaidet N, Newman SH, Hagemeijer W, Dodman T,‡ Cappelle J, Hammoumi S, et al, "Duck migration and past influenza A (H5N1) outbreak areas," *Emerging Infectious Disease*, July 2008, available at <http://www.cdc.gov/EID/14/7/1164 htm>

[29] Ibid.

birds, infected with highly pathogenic H5N1, died at the Qi nghai Lake nature reserve in central China. "Scientific stud ies comparing viruses from different outbreaks in birds have found that viruses from the most recently affected countries, all of which lie along migratory routes, are almost identical to viru ses recovered from dead migratory birds at Qinghai Lake."[30] Further, in a recen tly published study, a g roup of scien tists identified three distinct sublineages of H5N1 c irculating across Africa from 2006 to 2008. One of these sublineages can be traced back to the outbreak of H5N1 in m igratory waterfowl at China's Qinghai Lake in 2005.[31]

Figure 1. Waterfowl Flyways

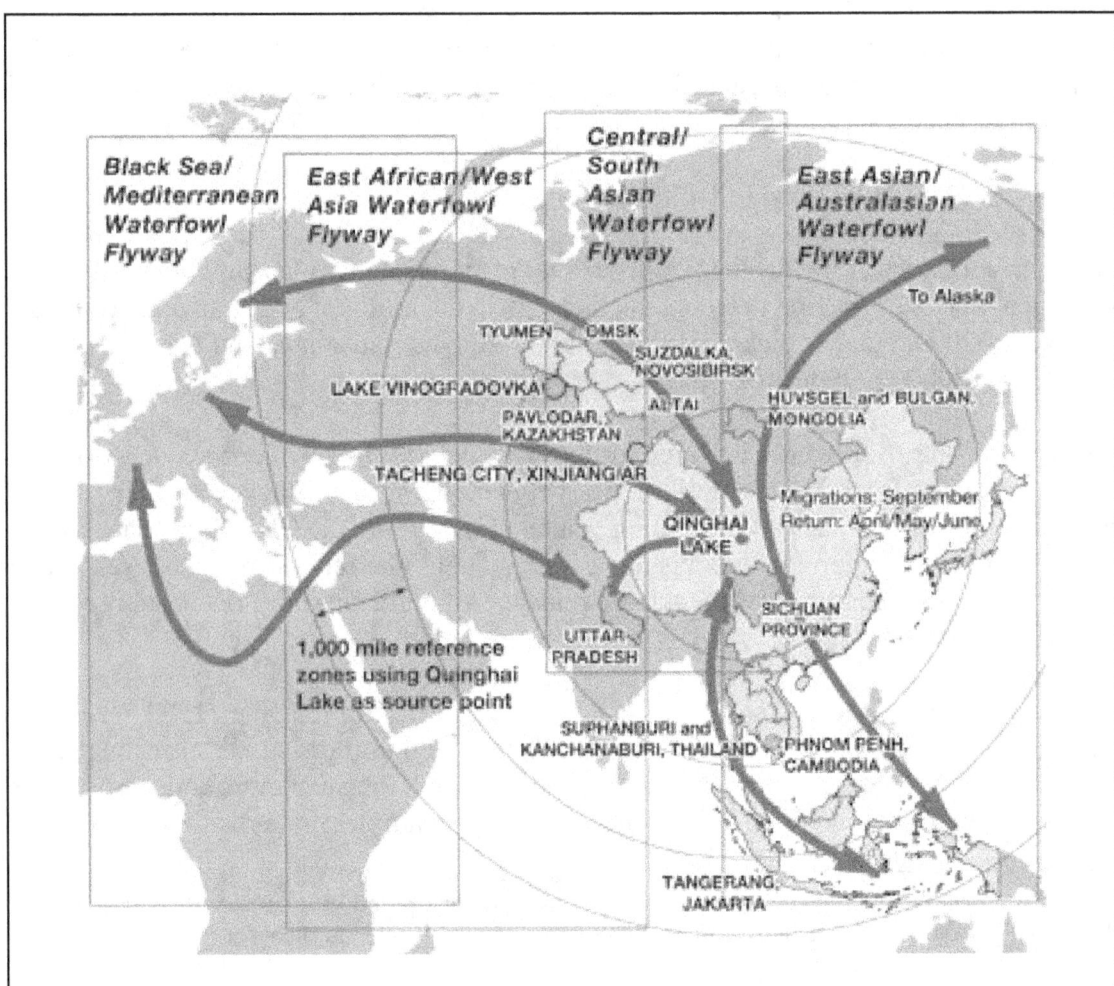

Many water birds (ducks, geese, swans) migrate between wetlands in the northern breeding areas and southern non-breeding areas, regularly crossing the borders of two or more countries. The birds can cover up to 1,000 miles per day . Source: World Food Pro gram Emergency Preparedness and Response Branch.

[30] World Health Organization, "Avian Influenza (bird flu): The Disease in Birds," February 2006, available at <http://www.who.int/mediacentre/factsheets/avian_influenza/en/#role>.
[31] Giovanni Cattoli, et al, "Highly Pathogenic Avian Influenza Virus Subtype H5N1 in Africa: A Comprehensive Phylogenetic Analysis and Molecular Characterization of Isolates," *PLoS*, March 2009, available at <http://www.plosone.org/article/info:doi/10.1371/journal.pone.0004842>.

Another possible way for the virus to circulate to countries not previously affected with H5N1 is through trade in poultry. Failure to use proper sanitation techniques and conduct inspections of the poultry could lead to the sale and distribution of infected poultry to new locations.

Nigeria is not the only African country aff ected by outbreaks of highly pathogenic avian H5N1. Since the initial outbreak in Nigeria in 2006, outbreak s have occurred in Benin, Burkina Faso, Ca meroon, Cote d'Ivoire, D jibouti, Egypt, Ghana, Niger, Sudan, and Togo.[32] Of the outbreaks of H5N1 in Africa, human cases of in fection have occurred in Djibouti, Nigeria, and Egypt. As of September 24, 2009, Egypt had reported 87 confirmed cases, with 27 fatali ties. In m any of these ca ses individuals infected with H5N1 had close contact with sick or dead poultry.[33]

H1N1 in Africa

Africa has also begun to report its first case s of pandem ic H1N1 influenza. 26 African countries have reported a to tal of 13,536 laboratory confir med cases of hum an infection with H1N1, including 75 deaths. [34] Countries that have developed, or begun developing pandemic H5N1 response plans will need to quickly adapt th e plans to resp ond to pandemic H1N1 before the virus spreads further into Africa. Weak health infrastructures, limited disease surveillance ca pabilities, and a whole host of underlying health issues such as large populations of HI V-infected individuals, will only exacerbate the potential devastating effects a serious H1N1 pandemic could have in Africa.

---

[32] World Organization for Animal Health, "Outbreaks of Avian Influenza (subtype H5N1) in poultry. From the end of 2003 to 11 April 2007, available at <http://www.oie.int/downld/AVIAN%20INFLUENZA/ Graph%20HPAI/graphs%20HPAI11_04_2007.pdf>.

[33] World Health Organization, "Avian influenza – situation in Egypt – update 23," September 24, 2009, available at <http://www.who.int/csr/don/2009_09_24/en/index html>.

[34] World Health Organization, Regional Office for Africa, "Pandemic (H1N1) 2009 in the African Region: Update 54," October 19, 2009, available at <http://www.afro.who.int/ddc/influenzaa/index.html>.

Nigeria: A Pandemic Planning Case Study

In recognition of the threat of an av ian influenza pandem ic, North Am erican Management, under contract to the Center for Technology and National Security Policy (CTNSP), developed and administered a program to help build pandemic influenza crisis-response capacities in Nigeria. The strategi c goal of CTNSP in providing this course of instruction was to work with the authors of the Nigerian National Integrated Avian and Pandemic Influenza Plan (National Plan) to assist them in defining an appropriate role for the Nigerian military in preserving national security during an influenza pandemic.

To achieve this aim , in June 2007, the project team developed a 4½-day Avian Influenza/Pandemic Influenza (AI/PI) Policy Planning workshop (see figure 2 for the curriculum). The Niger ian participants were representatives from the Departm ents of Agriculture, Health, and Inform ation, as well as m embers of the Pandem ic Influenza Control Center.

The primary focus of the workshop was to assist the attending Nigerian Ministerial officials in exercising and evaluating their nation's pandemic response plan, with the goal of furthering their understanding of potential national security im plications pandemic influenza could produce. A secondary goal was to understand the area of responsibility for military preparedness for pandemic influenza and ide ntify the range of detection, response, and containment roles the Nigerian military might be tasked to perform pre-pandemic, intra-pandemic, and post-pandemic.

Figure 2. Avian Influenza/Pandemic Influenza Policy Planning Course Curriculum

- Preparing for the Pandemic
    - Understanding the virus (discussion of H5N1 and the methods of transmission)
    - Communicating the risk: development of culturally relevant materials (strategic communication plan) for distribution to the population.
- Planning for the Pandemic
    - Assessing the national infrastructure (ability to maintain food availability and other essential services)
    - Identifying workforce availability and preparation of continuity of operations plans (COOP)
    - Developing medical and non-medical response plans
- Managing the Pandemic
    - All-day table-top exercise drawing on work of the previous three days
- After Action Review
    - Assessment of course objectives completion
    - Provide recommendation for follow on action plan, i.e. advanced Avian Influenza /Pandemic Influenza Senior Leadership Planning Course, Conference on Development of AI/PI National Response Plan

Analyzing the National Integrated Avian and Pandemic Influenza Plan

On June 13, 2007, eight of the workshop part icipants attended a "Technical Comm ittee" of the Nigerian AI/PI planning group. The purpose of the AI/PI planning group was to discuss the strengths and weaknesses of the Na tional Plan and suggest ways of filling in the gaps. T he authors of Nigeria's National Plan, primarily representatives from the Ministries of Health, Agriculture, and Infor mation, initially wanted to keep the working group to a sm all number by including only thos e entities that would, in their eyes, "add value to the process." T his definition lead to a planning group com posed exclusively of representatives from the Ministries of Agriculture, Health, and Information, and members of the Pandemic Influenza Control Center.

As a direct result of the program , the AI/PI planning group later identified a num ber of areas in which significant work was required to develop a full National Plan. Some of the most pressing areas included: the absence of specific roles for the Red Cross, non-governmental organizations (NGOs), and the Nigerian military, a lack of a national security perspective, a weak adm inistrative structure requiring strong agency "support plans," and the absence of decision points for declaring a state of emergency.

According to the sem inar participants, planning for the development of the new National Plan is one of the f irst times there has been extensive inter-ministry coordination. Normally, the m inistries work independently of one another, however, the AI/PI issue brought them together. Furthermore, the Nigeri an armed forces had been m entioned just once in the 72 pages of the March 22, 2007 dr aft of the National Plan. The workshop discovered that, until th e seminar, the issue of the military's role had n ot been carefully considered. The three departm ents (Agriculture, Health, and Inform ation) responsible for drafting the document agreed th at the m ilitary played an integ ral part of maintaining order in a peaceful democratic country and needed to be included in any future pandemic planning. When the participants returned in the afternoon to the workshop, they reported that the military and civil def ense organizations were f rom that poin t forward to be invited into the planning efforts.

While it was recognized that the National Plan is a fluid document, the participants stated that "you have to put your plan into action, even if it is incomplete;" and to "go with the plan you have and continuously revisit it. " It was the intention of the workshop participants to implement the current plan as it was and to continue to enhance it with the support of several of the m inistries that were not previously part of the initial planning process (i.e., Defense and Civil Defense).

The Value of the Military in Domestic Preparedness

The military's role in preparing for a pandemic can be defined as defending the nation by filling logistical gaps under the command of civilian authorities. The command structure under civilian authority was emphasized as the basis for success, particularly where communal conflict was occurring or expected.

In many countries, the military is considered the only institution capable of filling certain logistical roles (i.e., providing air transport, 24/7 security, mass distribution of key resources in multiple locations). Their ability to perform these functions is predicated on their being self-contained and self-sustaining. The military is uniquely able to rapidly deploy trained personnel, maintain an independent organized health care structure, and exercise unified command and control. Thus, the military can provide unparalleled resource allocation to civilian agencies through robust personnel, transportation, and communication capabilities, without being an additional burden to the civilian systems.

It is, therefore, imperative that Nigerian military representatives be involved in any future preparedness activities—specifically pandemic influenza exercises, participation in disaster response units, and the conduct of force health protection training. Based on discussions held during the June 2007 workshop in Nigeria, a list of proposed action items for the Ministry of Defense were identified:

- Assist civil response (Borders, Law Enforcement)
- Regulate poultry in barracks (Agriculture)
- Create awareness in barracks (Information)
- Poultry and human monitoring
- Report outbreaks to civilian authority through proper channels
- Request information that may impact military readiness
- Strengthen military health facilities (Health)
- Designate quarantine facilities on military bases

These planning functions were derived from the areas where the military would be involved in the *response* phase. In a severe pandemic event, typical support roles for the military would include operating in a single unified command structure under civilian leadership, providing command, control, and communications infrastructure, affording logistical assistance to first responder NGOs, including the Red Cross, and establishing a joint task force to coordinate efforts from all branches.

The most recent and updated version of the National Plan does a better job of incorporating the military into the planning process, however, their role is mentioned only briefly in the document and we recommend that it continue to be further expanded:

> In the early stages of pandemic emergence, the efforts of Government may be overwhelmed. It is envisaged that the armed forces, security agencies, and paramilitary forces (customs, immigration and prison officers) may be called upon to support pandemic containment activities at their source. They will then be called upon to provide vehicles, aircraft and operators to move personnel, equipment and supplies, as requested by the APIP&CC [Avian and Pandemic Influenza Prevention and Control Centre]; provide logistical support and air/ground transportation of disaster relief supplies, personnel and equipment; provide personnel and equipment for triage and emergency medical care and portable medical aid stations; provide space, as available to serve as resource

staging areas; and provide/and or coordinate traffic control and expedited routing for supply missions or personnel movements.[35]

Next Steps for Ministries of Health, Agriculture, and Information

In addition to th e drafting of an improved Nationa l Plan, every Ministry that was a member of the initia l Steering Committee and an author of the orig inal National Plan agreed to draft a Ministry Support Plan that would address the execution of each element of the National Plan from that Ministry's perspective. Utilizing the knowledge gained in the training seminar, each Ministry also agreed to draft their Support Plan with the role of the military in m ind. Further, a list of pr oposed action items for the Min istries of Agriculture, Health, and Information were identified. These action items provide a useful guide for other African countries in th e process of developing national pandem ic influenza response plans. They show the types of activities that shou ld be included in pandemic planning.

Ministry of Agriculture:
- Surveillance in poultry farms and markets
- Strengthen and enforce bio-security measures
- Frequent cleaning of poultry farms
- Strengthen regional laboratories to diagnose influenza subtypes
- Upgrade veterinary quarantine services at borders (equipment, training, etc.)
- Control movement of poultry and poultry products
- Register all poultry farms (locations, operations)
- Program for alternative livelihood (rehabilitation)
- Continue robust compensation program

Ministry of Health:
- Mobilize trained medical personnel
- Increase stockpiles of antivirals
- Develop protocols for access to stockpiles
- Standard operating procedures for pharmacological intervention
- Public personal protective measures and education
- Identify isolation facilities
- Active surveillance and contact tracing
- Health risk communication
- Activation of national and international health regulations

---

[35] Government of Nigeria, "Integrated National Avian and Pandemic Influenza Pandemic Influenza Response Plan 2007-2009," available at <http://nigeria.gov ng/NR/rdonlyres/44FA9DCA-AFEF-4C0E-8076-0C78984A175D/808/NIGERIAINTEGRATEDNATIONALAVIANAND PANDEMICINFLUENZA.pdf>.

Ministry of Information:

- Public information campaign and national press conference coordination with Agriculture, Health, and Defense
- Mobilize states' Ministry of Information for downstream information management
- Provision of public education via mass media coordination with Agriculture, Health, Defense, and Police
- Distribution of Information, Education, and Communication (IEC) materials (military and police support)
- Feedback mechanism coordination with NGOs, Community Based Organizations, (CBOs), and traditional rulers

According to the participants in the workshop, one of the most valuable lessons for them as a group was the newfound understanding of the importance of collaboration and communication between the various ministries. In a demonstration of this new paradigm, the ministries proposed a number of ways their agencies could collaborate. The participants identified opportunities to work cooperatively on issues such as the control of poultry movement and quarantine, ensuring continuity of the food supply, public education campaigns, medical waste management, carcass disposal, poultry culling oversight, capacity building for the military on AI/PI, activation of the command structure (Ministers, Governors), and conducting of simulations with participation from all stakeholders. Each of the above actions requires the involvement of a wide range of ministries, and their collaboration requires practiced interagency communication.

AFRICOM and Partnering for Public Health

"Improving the health infrastructure in   African nations is a 'productive and non-threatening' way to build stability on the continent"
- Dr. (Col) Schuyler Geller, Command Surgeon of U.S. Africa Command

On October 1, 2008, U.S. Africa Comm and (AFRICOM) was declared a fully unified command. One of six Department of Defe   nse regional military headquarters, AFRICOM's mission is to conduct sustained se curity engagement with African nations through military-to-military programs, military-sponsored activities, and other m ilitary operations as directed, to "create a stable   and secure African environm ent in support of U.S. foreign policy." [36] As part of its strategic obj   ectives, AFRICOM has identified protecting populations from deadly contagions, and in particular, deterring and containing pandemic influenza in Africa, as one of its priority objectives.

AFRICOM has stated that it views health as   a "bridge to peace and   security," and has developed an i mpressive number of health initiatives focused on Africa, including the Pandemic Response Program (PRP). In partnership with USAID, U.S. Pacific Command, and other international partners, such   as the W orld Food Program, AFRICOM is spearheading a m ulti-year pandemic response program aimed at stre ngthening partner African national military capabilities to respond to pandemic influenza in the contex t of larger national pandemic preparedness and resp onse plans. The PRP is part of the much broader USAID International Partnership on Avian and Pandem ic Influenza (IPAPI) effort aimed at enhancing global pandem ic preparedness. To date, USAID has already committed $543 million to international pandemic prevention and readiness issues. [37]

The PRP recognizes that national militaries have a critical role in health crisis response by providing logistical support for the transfer of food and medical supplies to pandemic-affected regions, protecting m edical staff, maintaining communications, and maintaining order and security in a time of uncertainty. [38] In an effort to assist African counties in the development of civil-military response plans, partners of the PRP will "train sen ior and mid-level military leaders in d isaster management and hum anitarian assistance, with a particular focus on pandem ic preparedness; to ensure that m ilitaries in ta rgeted 'pandemic preparedness' countries have deve   loped detailed plans of action directly supporting national plans; and to conduct exerci ses to test the im plementation of these plans and identify gaps or deficiencies." [39]

---

[36] AFRICOM, "Fact Sheet: AFRICOM Posture Statement: Ward Updates Congress on U.S. Africa Command," March 12, 2008, available at <http://www.africom mil/getArticle.asp?art=1799>.
[37] USAID, "Avian and Pandemic Influenza: Preparedness and Response," June 4, 2009, available at <http://www.usaid.gov/our_work/global_health/home/News/news_items/avian_influenza.html>.
[38] AFRICOM, "International Conference Focuses on Civil-Military Influenza Pandemic Response Plans," May 19, 2009, available at <http://www.africom mil/getArticle.asp?art=3030>.
[39] Ibid.

The PRP comes at a vital time in pandemic influenza planning. With the recent WHO declaration of an H1N1 pandemic, many African nations need immediate assistance in the development of civil and military pandemic response plans. During an influenza pandemic it is estimated that up to 40 percent of an organization's staff may be absent at any time. For a nation that is already hosting a large population of immuno-compromised individuals—such as an African nation with high rates of HIV or AIDS patients—the absenteeism rate will likely sky rocket. As a result, an influenza pandemic may be most devastating in fragile democracies where stability is constantly in jeopardy. These states are significant due to their vulnerability and the consequently greater need for them to develop a strong action plan. To be most effective in preserving a state's human capital, preparations for an influenza pandemic must focus on the readiness issue—particularly in a state with a medical establishment that will assuredly not be able to handle the stresses created by a pandemic.[40] An international presence, such as is being developed by the AFRICOM PRP, may be helpful in preventing an untoward outcome by assisting in the development of a contingency plan and thorough training of military personnel to ensure its execution.[41]

---

[40] Robert Armstrong et al., "Weathering the Storm: Leading Your Organization Through a Pandemic," Defense and Technology Paper 38 (Washington, DC: Center for Technology and National Security Policy, November 2006), available at <http://www ndu.edu/CTNSP/Def_Tech/DTP%2038% 20Weathering%20The%20Storm.pdf>.

[41] One potential partner outside of African national militaries for the PRP to engage with is the Economic Community of West African States (ECOWAS). Founded in 1975, ECOWAS is a regional group of fifteen West African countries. Among the agencies under ECOWAS is the West African Health Organization (WAHO). Civilian components under the PRP, such as USAID, could potentially engage with WAHO in pandemic preparedness planning for governments in Africa, thus ensuring national governments and militaries have cohesion in their planning.

Conclusion

In the opinion of the participants from the various Nigerian Ministries and the Nigerian military, the workshop "was a huge success. " However, they also reco gnized that the interdependencies they discovered throughout the workshop need further refinem ent and assignment of responsibility. In recognition of these lingering deficiencies, many participants requested additional training in their post-workshop comments.

A further concern of the participants in th e training workshops was the universal belief that a "pandem ic knows no boundaries." The National Integrated Avian and Pandem ic Influenza Plan Steering Comm ittee members have addressed, and will continue to r efine through their respective agency s upport plans, the issues of bo rder control in the event of a pandemic incident. However, they were concerned that their neighboring countries have not developed plans or strategies to addre ss a pandemic. To support the integrity of the National Integrated Avian and Pandem ic Influenza Plan, it is essential to provide sim ilar training to border countries a nd the guidance necessary to operationalize each of their national pandemic plans.

The unresolved concerns of the Nigerian participants present an opportunity for AFRICOM and its P andemic Response Program partners to help selected A frican partners build their pandem ic response capabil ities. The recent decl aration of an H1N1 pandemic demonstrates the urgent necessity for countries to have pandem ic response plans in place and the necessi ty for continued international aid resources devoted to assisting our partner nations in pandemic response planning and mitigation.

www.ingramcontent.com/pod-product-compliance
Lightning Source LLC
Chambersburg PA
CBHW082032190526
45166CB00017B/3444